Hospital Survival

A personal, serious, metaphysical and occasionally humorous examination of surviving a serious disease.

Jay E. Morrow

authorHOUSE®

AuthorHouse™
1663 Liberty Drive
Bloomington, IN 47403
www.authorhouse.com
Phone: 1-800-839-8640

First published by AuthorHouse 12/9/2009

ISBN: 978-1-4490-1094-2 (e)
ISBN: 978-1-4490-1095-9 (sc)
ISBN: 978-1-4490-1096-6 (hc)

Printed in the United States of America
Bloomington, Indiana

This book is printed on acid-free paper.

Contents

During 2008, my fifty fourth year, I nearly died three times, died once, was fired, and spent almost as many months in the hospital as I spent at home. In many ways this is my attempt to exorcize the demons that I created that year as well as warn others of what they can expect when they enter a hospital. In many cases, this is either humorous or terrifying. I hope that I bring perspective of these issues out into the open.

The Cruise from Hell:

Now my wife is one of the great joys of my life. She loves to travel, plan travel and eat well. We decided to take a short cruise along the southern California coast just for fun and give me time to decompress and relax. We planned to take a cruise from LA to Santa Catalina, San Diego, and Ensenada and get back to LA over a short week. We would leave on a Sunday and get back on Friday. Prior to our catching a plane from Seattle to Los Angeles, she planned on meeting with her group of divas (a local women's group) to have fun and disparage the male gender. Since I think I am male (Last time I checked) I didn't want to cramp their style or become an object of ridicule. It was very plain that my presence was not only not needed, it was not desired. After a long workweek, I was feeling a little rundown but took this as an opportunity to play a little poker at our local Native American casino, with the goal of earning additional money for the trip.

Usually when I play poker, it's for several hours. I am known as a very shrewd player that normally is tough for my competitors to figure out. That night I was up by $100 dollars within an hour and this would normally increase my desire to win even more, but I decided to call it a night and head home. For some reason, I just felt "off' and as any true player knows, this can lead to a disaster at any poker table. I cashed in my chips and headed home. I arrived to find our little driveway still packed with the "diva's" cars. Not wanting to create any type of scene I pulled down onto another road and went to sleep in our comfortable van.

I awoke with the local Sheriff shining a light into my eyes. He wanted to know if I was drunk or casing out a neighborhood house for a burglary. Once I explained the situation he let me go, but I could tell that he was going to come around regularly to ensure that I was not some "ne-r do well". I called home and my wife said I should come home and crash in my daughter's old bedroom while she continued with her group. (my daughter was away at college at the time). When I arrived, I got the usual good natured catcalls from the divas, went downstairs and fell fast asleep in the bed. I awakened just as the last diva left. I crawled into my own bed and went fast asleep again.

We left early the next morning to go to the airport and catch our flight to LA. Once again, I felt "off", like I was coming down with the flu, but I didn't have any fever, nausea, or upper respiratory issues. All I had was a feeling that something was not right.

The flight to LA was uneventful, but rather than meeting my wife's friend in LA, we just went to the hotel and crashed. I got in some reading and watched some TV while my wife swam in the hotel pool; and once again fell fast asleep. Still I had no symptoms other than a general malaise and lack of energy. In retrospect, I should have been more in tune with my body's signals and realized that I was ill and rapidly approaching a critical phase. But you know how it is, it didn't seem like anything I hadn't dealt with before.

The next day, we got up early, had the hotel breakfast, and headed off to the cruise terminal. But, my left hip hurt enough that I was starting to drag it when I was rolling my bag. As usual, it took standing in four different lines to just get close to the cruise ship. This is like waiting for your driver's license, as you find that this line is not the right one and you must go to station B and please bring the appropriate forms... I was really not feeling well, but my wife made me promise not to say anything. Cruise ships were known to deny boarding to customers showing signs of the flu. This is to protect both the cruise ship personnel and the other passengers. Both the cramped quarters and ventilating systems can lead to a fast spreading respiratory ailment.

While we were waiting in the next line to allow us through to security, my wife swears that she could smell the odor of ammonia surrounding me. I was more concerned with the hip pain, worrying that I had sciatica. Finally we had our IDs generated, our pictures taken and were attending one of the ubiquitous buffets for lunch. I could not move on my left leg without hopping or dragging the entire leg. When my wife left to explore the ship, I went below to our cabin and crashed again. Once again ignoring many danger signals. Little did I know that this was the last day I would walk for over a year.

When dinner call was sounded, I passed and watched a movie in our cabin. One I would see over 8 times in the next three days. I was already seriously overweight, but now I found that I was retaining an alarming amount of fluid and weighed well over 280 pounds. Trying to shove my enormous bulk around a tiny cabin became a nightmare of shuffling, tripping over bags, and just generally moving in slow motion.

The next morning, we anchored off of Santa Catalina. But the pain condition had grown worse. I asked my wife to take me to the ships sickbay. There were nothing but low chairs and I had the feeling that if I wasn't diagnosed with seasickness, I was not going to get much help. After waiting for at least a half hour, I met with a Doctor who spoke at best broken English (I later found out he was Ukrainian). After a quick examination, he thought it might be sciatica. A nice little Filipino nurse came in and gave me possibly the most painful shot I have ever received. They pumped me full of muscle relaxers and morphine. I think they loaded me up with these drugs to get me out of the way, and not to give me a cure. This was my first experience with morphine, but certainly not my last over the next months. Filled with morphine, I was amazed to find out that the painted landscapes in our cabin were full of funny and talkative people who thought my every thought was hilarious. In other words I was hallucinating.

For the next three days, I got progressively worse, despite increasing dosages of morphine. The space in our cabin, which was roughly the size of a broom closet with a shower, grew smaller with the addition of a wheelchair. I was introduced to another doctor, this one was Costa Rican. During frequent visits to sickbay, I could hear the two doctors arguing my case in several different languages. My two main memories were the young Filipino nurse that gave injections which I came to think of as a form of torture and the individuals that kept stepping out of the landscape paintings in our cabin and discussing poker with me. I recognized that things were getting very bad, when my wife returned from Catalina with an extra-large t-shirt that did not even come close to covering my enormous girth. This highlighted for both my wife and I that something seriously was wrong with me. While I was working my way through my own private hell, my wife was dealing with the ship's medical staff. They had decided that I should be put ashore as soon as possible. Although they had a complete sickbay and operating room, I think this decision was mainly based on avoiding the serious negative publicity of having a tourist die on board. Not only would this have been a negative outcome for me personally, but could affect the cruise ships marketing for some time.

My wife, bless her soul, knew that having me in a Mexican hospital was not in my best interests. She demanded that I stay on board ship an additional day to get me back to LA. She also got the ship's doctors to write an emergency transport letter to get me to an emergency room as soon as possible. This would get me priority seating on any flights necessary to get me home. Luckily, the Costa Rican doctor not only wrote the letter, but he had noticed that throughout my entire trip, I had had a slightly elevated temperature. As a precaution he prescribed a general antibiotic, this was to make sure I made it to LA before I died. Once again, in retrospect, this probably saved my life. Calling a friend of my wife's in LA and enlisting her aid, we were able to just barely make the terminal to catch the only flight open from LA to Seattle. Without her friend's help, we would never have been to take the various back-roads that shave minutes off the travel time from the cruise terminal to the airport.

Next came the rush through the terminal. I was so loaded with morphine, by this time, the trip remains a blur. Alaska Airlines would not give us a wheelchair until we got a boarding pass. Knowing every moment counted, my wife and her friend, Claudia pulled out all the stops and managed to get not only the wheelchair, but grabbed an Alaska airlines attendant who also got a boarding pass for me without standing in line. I vaguely remember going through security, (most people already know how much fun this is, when you are well). The TSA staff took my bag and handled it separately, while the attendant rushed me to the gate. My wife sat down and for the first time in several days let out a sigh of relief. She was talking to the other passengers, when she turned to me and asked "Where's your bag?" In my drug induced stupor, my only response was "What bag?" My wife took off at a run to return on the concourse to security. She yelled back to me to have them hold the plane. I rolled the wheelchair over to the gate attendant and in a semi-coherent fashion I finally got across to her that my wife had returned to security for my bag. As they were just about to close the doors, my wife showed up at a trot. We were the last ones on the plane.

I assume that I slept the whole way back; at least I don't recall any passage of time. My next semi-coherent memory is a trip up I-5 from the airport to ABC Hospital. ABC is one of the premier diagnostic hospitals on the west coast. Throughout the car trip (Meant both as a means of travel and my body's altered state due to the morphine) the signs seemed to be expanding as I looked at them. It was like they were popping in a non-continuous fashion. As soon as I looked at them, they expanded to twice or four times their original size. In some ways, deep down inside of my brain, I was fascinated by the effect. I was almost disappointed when we arrived at the exit and pulled into the emergency area of the hospital. For the first time, but certainly not the last, I was asked one of the most nonsensical and finally irritating questions that I would hear over the next ten days "Can you walk or do you need some help?" My mom met us there, while the intricacies of our insurance were discussed. My Mom would become one of my main advocates during the next year. I sat in the lobby for three hours alternating between hallucinations and reality. Actually, I preferred the hallucinations, since in reality I was sinking deeper into septicemia (More on this later). I watched several idiots come in to the same area. Even when not on drugs, I find the emergency room waiting area in a major metropolitan hospital to be one of the most unintentionally humorous places in our modern world. A good comedian could get three acts, just by observing the situations that arrive. The TV series when they are not romanticized are not far from the truth. One situation involved a young adult that had questioned the manhood of several huge individuals from a neo-Nazi bar. When he came arrived, he seemed to be bleeding from a multitude of cuts to his head and chest. I was finally admitted to the hospital at around 6:00 PM that night, after arriving at 3:00 PM. By 7:00 PM I was surrounded by a cadre of approximately ten doctors. This was the first time I heard 'septicemia".

1st Recipe for disaster:

1. Develop a medically interesting disease
2. Be in foreign country and not be conversant in the native language
3. Be misdiagnosed
4. Have no network to understand what was on-going in a potentially life threatening situation

If my wife had not told the cruise sickbay personnel that we would not be getting off in Mexico, or had delayed in any way getting me back to the hospital, I am positive that I would have succumbed to the disease I now carried.

The way I was:

Prior to 2008, I was always the type of individual that needed to work to somehow validate my existence. During my summer breaks from college, I would work 60-70 hours/week for $1.75 an hour plus a potential end of season bonus. This coupled with a tuition scholarship allowed me to pay for probably 60-70% of my college costs. My parents would call up and offer $15 occasionally, which I was always deathly afraid of taking. I knew how hard they both worked to save money and I was totally averse to living off of their subsidies. Even when I changed majors from Oceanography to Chemistry I refused to waste the credits I had already earned. So, I got two degrees, one in Chemistry and one in Oceanography.

Sometime during the next thirty years, I found time to have two kids that we put through college. Our oldest daughter has fraternal twins and seems to be carrying on our tradition of overachievement.

When I graduated from college on June 11, 1977 I already had a job starting on June 13. I spent the next thirty years working an average of 50-60 hours per week. I was epitome of the workhorse of American industry, the backbone at the end of the baby boomer generation. I moved into management in 1980 and was the example of the driven manager that believed, I should outwork the workforce. If they started at 7, I was there at 6:30. I rarely took more than 1 day off to be sick and had to be told to take vacations. This worked fine for the first thirty years, but it led to overwork, bad diets, stress, and ultimately the realization that I could become ill from my approach to life. It is a fouled up and neurotic approach to living life. It is designed so that when you die, your family is wealthy. Something that I was well on the road to achieving without even checking with them, that this is what they wanted.

The first manifestation was the arrival of too much weight, which led to a diagnosis of type 2 diabetes. After being treated for three years with metformin, I was found to have developed anemia. My heart (Thank Goodness) was fine and thanks to my genetics so was my blood pressure (120 over 75), but I was still seriously overweight, stressed and was sent from one specialist to another concerning the anemia. The initial diagnosis indicated that I needed a liver biopsy. My ultrasound had showed initial signs of fatty liver and an enlarged spleen. In other words, I had developed cirrhosis of the liver without the fun of drugs or alcohol.

Now my first example of what to expect in the future; my liver doctor met me again six months later and wanted to schedule an ultrasound. I pointed out that I had already had an ultrasound, he argued that he never received the results. Since it was done in his office, I found this too difficult to accept and that I did not care for doctors that would not admit errors or procedural problems. After all I was a management professional that had hundreds of people working with me. We occasionally made mistakes, why shouldn't the medical profession.

In addition, I did not care for this particular doctor's bedside manner, and found another doctor, the best on the west coast that stated that I didn't need a biopsy. He diagnosed that I had NASH (Non-Alcoholic Steato Hepatitis). He also said that well over 20% of the type 2 Diabetics were developing this new add-on to the disease. This is a new development in the diabetic community and should be more publicized to everyone involved. After consulting with my internist they moved me off metformin and onto glypicide, which appears to be deal with the liver better. Immediately, my blood test results were under much better control. I believed that I was in control of the situation and just needed to lose more weight. When I was in college, my weight was 170 pounds, and at this point in time I weighed 80 pounds more than I should. It dawned on me that changes in my diet of carbohydrates (I love pasta), more relaxation, and an increase in physical activity were definitely indicated, if I planned on seeing my family in the future.

Septicemia and Encephalopathy:

Back to the events and infections that so affected me over the next twelve months. I was diagnosed with Septicemia, which is a serious, life-threatening infection that gets worse very quickly. It can arise from infections throughout the body, including infections in the lungs, abdomen, and urinary tract. It may come before or at the same time as infections of the bone, central nervous system, or other tissues. It can begin with spiking fevers, chills, rapid breathing, and rapid heart rate. The person, in this case me, looks very ill.

The symptoms rapidly progress to shock with decreased body temperature (hypothermia), falling blood pressure, confusion (Something I rarely experienced during my previous fifty four years), other changes in mental status, and blood clotting problems that lead to a specific type of red spots on the skin. It is a serious condition that requires hospital treatment. Anyone infected may be end up in an intensive care unit (ICU) very quickly. Septic shock has a high death rate, exceeding 50%, depending on the type of disease organism involved and how quickly the patient is hospitalized will normally determine the outcome. Septicemia is not common but it is devastating. Early recognition may prevent progression to shock.

After arriving at hospital ABC, the entire hospital seemed to be geared to finding me a cure. The doctors were particularly concerned that my heart could have become infected. Now in the hospital, there are many dedicated professionals who care greatly for you and want you to get well. This dedication and care covers up many flaws in the overall system. These professionals are held in check by an army of administrators and clerks, who want to ensure that the services provided are paid, preferably up front. The technical side was serious about relieving my body of the tremendous load of fluid (I now weighed over 300 pounds, much of it retained fluid), but also locating the original source of the infection. Because of the continual loads of morphine, I spent much of my time speaking to another cast of characters coming out of a fresh series of landscapes. Sometimes these people would even play poker with me. This caused great interest throughout my family, as I would occasionally look away from their conversation to tell someone that I was raising their poker hand. In addition, if someone tried to talk with me, I would just drift off to sleep in mid-sentence. Since I arrived with a mysterious infection from Mexico, I was isolated; and the potential need for an operation, kept me from receiving any food, including ice chips. My mouth became like a desert.

I had developed some very strange symptoms:

- I would sleep during the day and be up all night
- I could not concentrate on any reading material
- I smelled of ammonia (According to my wife)
- I was hallucinating
- My wrists and hands would flap uncontrollably (Kind of like a wounded seagull)

Given my general symptoms, the doctors decided that I also had encephalopathy. Hepatic encephalopathy leads to changed cognitive function. This can range from subtle deficits in higher mental functions (in mild cases) to coma (in severe cases). Left untreated, severe hepatic encephalopathy can cause death. One more fear to ad to my ponderings in my drugged late night hours. I apologize for the technical terms in the next few pages, but it is important to understand what was happening to me at the time.

Manifestations of hepatic encephalopathy can be "day-night reversal." I prefer the more laymen's term of "Vampirism", since it evokes a different image than that of a sick and helpless person. In other words, affected individuals tend to sleep during the day and stay awake at night. (Thank goodness there is no coffin involved). Another early manifestation is impairment in spatial perception. This can be made apparent by noting the patient's poor ability to copy or draw various simple images, e.g., cube, star, or clock. This deficit can also be demonstrated by administering a test that has the patient connect a number of randomly-placed dots on a sheet of paper (the "trail test" or "numbers connecting test").

Virtually any metabolic disturbance may precipitate hepatic encephalopathy. Infection is an important precipitant of hepatic encephalopathy. In some cases, the only clinical manifestation of the infection is the development of the encephalopathy. In fact, this is a frequent phenomenon in patients whose ascites has become infected (i.e., spontaneous bacterial peritonitis). In laymen's terms my body cavity was filling up with fluid providing a perfect growth medium for dangerous infections.

Although I was only semi-coherent, I overheard several discussions amongst my doctors that believed that my heart and lungs were infected. It was finally decided that I would need an MRI scan to determine the truth. Both my mom and my wife began to question some of the treatments and decisions being made. For example the MRI looked at only my heart and lungs and did not closely examine my stomach or hip. Luckily they did manage to wrestle my cell phone away from me, so I wouldn't call anyone in my business or family circle of any importance and piss them (unnecessarily) off. To say the least, I wasn't at my most mentally acute. At least that's what my family told me later.

At some point Transport arrived in my room to take me to the MRI imaging area with the usual question "Can you walk?" I must admit to my sarcastic side responding to that question in what can only be described as a caustic response. When I identified that I could not, we had to wait for the additional 4 people necessary to move me onto the gurney for movement to the MRI facility. We moved out through the labyrinth of halls elevators, and waysides. I began to think of the early days when I took trips on a train only to be on a siding while the express rumbled by. We arrived at MRI facility, where once again I heard "Can you walk?" I hope you are beginning to see why this question was beginning to upset me. Okay I will admit, I'm not an easy going guy in some situations but the hospital staff has their share of blame on this issue.

Keep in mind that the imaging technicians in the hospital are the flakes of hospital staff, see the examples below. Not only are they not medical, they do not really understand how the imaging works. They have been trained to take pictures of you. As an example, an MRI technician dropped some popcorn in the facility. Without thinking, they brought in a vacuum cleaner. The vacuum cleaner is metallic, while the main guts of the MRI equipment is a huge electromagnet. When the vacuum clanged onto the MRI machine (M stands for magnetic) it only caused $300,000 in damage. I'm sure that's in my bill someplace. Okay maybe not my part of my direct bill but certainly part of medical costs for all of us. A small price to pay to pick up a few kernels of popcorn. Another situation, which may be an urban legend, was the requirement for an armed policeman to be in attendance when a felon was scanned. His gun although holstered dragged him into the machine and pinned him to the side. They had to pry him off. The technicians put me into the tunnel with headphones so I could hear the instructions and listen to a rock station on the radio. At many points, I was supposed to hold my breath. Unfortunately the technician forgot to tell me when I could take another breath. I almost passed out.

At the first break, I told them that I was pretty tired of hearing the radio commercials and they could just turn off the radio. The orderly turned them off. Unfortunately they also turned off my ability to hear the instructions such as when I was supposed to hold my breath, etc. Now imagine being in long snake-like tube trying to hold your breath. I didn't start out claustrophobic, but I was rapidly getting more and more frightened. Instead of being done in a half an hour, as I'd been briefed, they finally noticed their mistake and we were done in an hour and a half. If I hadn't been so doped up on morphine, I am sure that the tube would have had a bulge in it where I would have bounced off of it trying to get out. When the doctors reviewed the test, they found that I had so much fluid retained they couldn't see anything of importance. So the first test was a complete waste of time.

Within the day, I was loaded up on more drugs and then had a group of doctors sticking me with syringes to draw off as much excess fluid as possible. This, they hoped would allow a useful MRI. I do recall hearing the phrase that "this wouldn't hurt a bit." HAH! Imagine having a five inch long needle directed into your stomach. Do you think it might hurt even just a little? Since no one explained how this might hurt or what was involved when they stuck a the five inch needle in your my stomach, my addled mind created its own scenario for what was happening to me. This was my first experience with a metaphysical component of operations. None of the doctors told me what was involved, so my mind convinced me that I been moved to a local park and medical students were practicing on my immobile body. I was sequestered in the trees and I couldn't talk. It was like being imprisoned in your own body undergoing unusual medical experiments (Twilight Zone music, please). I felt if I could only raise my head I would be able to see the hospital from the operating table through the parks trees. My mental acuity at this point was almost non-existent. My family was worried that I was making less and less sense, and they were treating me more and more like a child, with simple instructions and the removal of any dangerous equipment such as cell phones or glasses.

The operation to try and aspirate the fluid was both painful and a complete failure. Very little fluid was removed from my system. The doctors decided on a much less invasive technique, where I would be loaded up with antibiotics to combat the infection and diuretics to remove the fluid. One thing did occur, when they attempted to aspirate my hip, they scraped the bone and found an infection. When this infection was cultured, it was determined to be staph (possibly MRSA- the flesh eating variety). They began immediate treatments with heavy duty antibiotics. It wasn't until much later that I understood the limitations associated with this kind of treatment. (Since they had not discovered the source of the infection, there was the chance that they would miss the underlying cause of my disease.) The addition of lactulose meant that I had now been given a laxative without any ability to move to bathroom. This meant many a panicked call to the nursing staff for assistance, always without time to get to the bathroom.

2ⁿᵈ Recipe for Disaster

- Take one patient unable to walk
- Feed them a laxative
- Watch the area between the bathroom and the bed for surprises
- Laugh outside of the room

And Now for Something Completely Different:

This was made famous by Monty Python's Flying Circus, and it is a good time to deviate from a chronological telling of this story to some common things that you will find in every hospital.

- **The night nurse:**
  There is nothing to compare to the inherent power of the night nurse. The closest that it can be understood is the role of an eighteenth century sea captain traveling on the other side of the earth. They will brook no mutinies or even questioning of their decisions, without serious repercussions. This can be as simple as not responding to the call button, withholding painkillers, to the sudden and inexplicable need to insert a catheter. That is not to say that I have not met many dedicated people or that I would want the responsibilities of their position. Hospital Administrators rarely provide enough support to these caring people, so they must be tough.

- **Transport:**
  The need to go the bathroom, move to the operating room or to the MRI room is always accompanied by the arrival of a short underweight orderly, whose first question is "Can you stand up and walk?" This can become increasingly irritating when it is obvious that you cannot in anyway stand up.

- **The statement, "This won't hurt a bit":**
  You should be aware that his won't be hurting them, but is necessary for your overall improvement. Each time I heard it, it hurt like hell. Pain is a way for your body to tell you things are not right, so any unexplained pain may be an infection. As I stated earlier, we as a society usually ignore these signals and try to power through the pain. Subsequently infections are almost always associated with syringes, scalpels, or catheters.

- **Doctor's demeanor:**
  Heaven help you if you are designated as an "Interesting Medical Case". This is always accompanied by at least two additional doctors who need to show off to their colleagues how smart they are. They begin by discussing how grave and complex your condition is and what they would do to fix it.

- **Sleep:**
  Forget about any kind of restful and life sustaining sleep in a hospital. It is vitally important (I Guess) that your vital signs be taken every two hours. Systematically, a nurse arrives just as you have finally achieved sleep to

wake you up. She will take your temperature and blood pressure, and then disappear for another two hours, murmuring that you should try and get some sleep. This is just about enough time for you to go back to sleep. Also, it is guaranteed that the only thing on TV is infomercials concerning how you can sue your medical staff for giving you the wrong medications. (Something to think about late at night in the hospital)

- **How to get from location to location:**
Because of the growth of the medical industry, hospitals have expanded in a haphazard fashion that means to get from point A to point B, requires the use of three separate elevators and stops in several hallways to transfer you to the new areas responsibilities. Each of these will use the term "Can you stand and walk?"

- **Your chart:**
If you stay in the hospital for any length of time, your chart will grow astronomically. Usually this growth is approximately two inches for every week. Although the course of treatment is occasionally consulted by the nursing staff and team of doctors, most of the time, it is simply used to ensure that you have not the slightest idea of what is in your chart or how that affects your treatment. Unless, you are especially vigilant or aware it is used by all of the nurses to tell you what the doctor ordered, whether he ordered it or not. I am diabetic and have a liver condition, yet hardly anyone ever made sure that I did not receive glucose drips or

avoided aspirin, acetaminophen or ibuprofen. If I or my advocate (More on this later) didn't catch it, I could receive many different and dangerous prescriptions. A chart is incredibly detailed and maintained with notations at every visit by someone on staff. With the amount of data available here it is confounding that it is read so little while written in so much. Sometimes I wonder if it is to be used for treatment or accumulating data to ward against adverse actions.

- **The Bed:**

The bed in a hospital is designed to keep you inside and not allow you to control this aspect of your life. At least 50% of the bed's in which I slept did not work. Sometimes the controls in one direction would work, while it would never work in the other direction. I could raise my feet, but not lower them. There I would be with my feet in the air, not able to stand up on my own and a bed that malfunctioned in the lower feet mode. So It was kind a of a dead end alley, where you would end up in totally weird positions without any way to return the bed to a normal position. Universally, this made me look like a complete fool to the orderly, whose controls always worked. But being confined to the bed I could not reach his controls.

- **The TV:**

TVs never work in the hospital. There is no guide channel, nor information on what is currently playing. If they do work, it is impossible to figure out the channels.

If you do change the channels, you will never find the same channel again. Not only that, but the staff in the hospital could care less if they work or don't work, even though this is often your only method of keeping your mind from stressing out on your condition. However it is guaranteed that you can receive every infomercial known to man. I confess that many of them caught my attention, concerning how to get help in suing for malpractice. Now I occasionally would look at some of these with the idea, that the hospital could really use them. The sham wow to pick up spills, or oxy-clean to remove those ugly stains. Thankfully, I kept these ideas to myself, which probably kept me out of the psychiatric ward.

- **Timing:**

The absolute lowest ebb of any patient in the hospital is late at night. You are emotionally drained, scared, angry and sometimes confused at a time when few answers or physicians are available. This also is the time, when services are minimal and usually when your advocate is not allowed to be around.

- **Continuity, or lack thereof:**

Most of your care in the hospital is provided by a core of dedicated professional nurses. They are mostly well trained and considerate of your feelings. Unfortunately, because of scheduling, as soon as you get used to one team (Usually a registered nurse, a certified nurse practitioner, and an orderly) the team changes. This means all of time spent building a rapport with the first team is completely lost and you have to start over again. Rapport is important so they can trust when you feel abnormal and you can trust them to respond adequately. I would just reach a relationship with team, when shift change would occur and an entire new set of personalities would be involved. New personnel may take hours or days to decide that you are not a complainer by nature and that something should be done.

New Developments
& Old Situations:

At night, I had interesting dreams or hallucinations that made my life fun and at the same time terrifying. One of my most enduring memories was that I became a complete existensionalist mote. The walls, floor, and ceiling of the hospital disappeared. I was stretched out and floating through the blackness of the universe. My body vibrated with energy as if I were multiple versions of the same person. I was seeing myself cascade across the sky with multiple copies floating through space or a deck of cards fanned across the sky. Whatever I thought of happened as soon as I thought of it. The stars and planets seemed to float by as I moved through the cosmos. It seemed as if my body was vibrating like a bow string. I could stretch out my hands and move a planet aside or wave my hands and stir the stars like the phosphorescence in a pool of sea water. The power and feelings were almost overwhelming. Nothing existed unless I made it so. My mind processes speeded up to the point where I could not always follow the experiences. Later, when I tried to bring about the same effect, I was a dismal failure. In fact, I think I peed all over myself. That definitely removed any godlike tendencies.

Now, keep in mind that in real life, I was living in a small town, with no building more than one story high. I hallucinated that I had been restrained in a facility six stories high and was being farmed for pharmaceuticals to assist our troops in Iraq. I felt that I had not been consulted, so I began removing these tubes that had been installed (Kind of like the scene from the Matrix). Before the hospital noticed, I was bleeding from multiples sites. It turned out that my removal of tubes, was real and not a hallucination. Now the nursing staff could not find a vein of sufficient magnitude to get me the antibiotics I needed. Luckily, they called in a specialist who must have been the Daniel Boone of the hospital, because he found a good vein in my left hand. This illustrates what would happen every evening in my mind, in that I would awaken in a room that seemed to bear no resemblance to where I was during the day, and that the nursing staff never seemed to understand what was happening to me each night. The nursing staff had no visibility to my inner life, so they just thought they could tell me not to do something. I would listen attentively and then at night when the visions would reassert themselves, I would do what the visions told me to do.

As I became increasingly desperate to get some fluids, food or even ice, I overheard discussions between two factions of doctors. The orthopedic surgeons wanted to operate and open up the hip to find the infection. The infection specialists wanted to find out the underlying cause without invading the hip. While this discussion was occurring, I was not getting any food. This is my first survival of death, since they prescribed a heavy glucose IV. (Not exactly the right choice for a diabetic.) This occurred during one of my more coherent moments, so I was able to call attention to this salient fact. My advocates also caught them at least twice trying to give me the same heavy duty glucose. Finally they marked both the doorway and the chart with "Do not feed or give glucose". (Like Yellowstone-Do not feed the bears!!!)

This was also mimicked to a lesser degree by the habit of reducing pain medication by using acetaminophen products in conjunction with morphine or oxycotin. This is directly contrary in how to deal with liver issues, since acetaminophen should not be given to liver compromised patients. Although this was already identified in my chart, it would still be prescribed on occasion. It just highlights that charts are consulted only rarely and usually only for the last few days. This situation with acetaminophen occurred on an additional three times. Each time either I or my advocates caught it before it was administered. It draws attention to one of the most common mistakes that occur in hospitals, the inadvertent use of the wrong medication. Transfer of patient information between nursing shifts usually do not use the patient charts but are rather based more on personal discussions between the two shifts.

A typical conversation with all of the doctors and my family would go as follows:

Doctor1:   Are you in pain?

Me: Yes, but I mainly can't talk and am really hungry or thirsty.

Doctor 2:   We may have to operate.

Doctor 3:   We shouldn't give any food or drink.

Head Nurse: We posted a sign not to give any food.

My wife: You closed your eyes, were you asleep?

Me: I am just tired of being sick.

My Wife: It sounded like you were snoring

Doctor 2:   We could fix the snoring issue, if we operate.

Doctor 3:   Should we operate?

Doctor 1:   We don't know where the infection started from, so why would we operate.

My wife: You closed your eyes again.

Me: (To myself, it seemed better than talking to the two people who just walked out of the painting.) I am listening to them discuss my case.

My wife: I think you were sleeping.

Me: It has about the same effect, since no one will give me any ice chips.

| Doctor 2: | We need to run a few more tests. Can you walk? |
| Me: | Snoring loudly....... |

Repeat this conversation, several times per day for their full effect.

One of the many intriguing phenomena would be how my hospital room would change at night in my mind. Awakened for my vital signs, I would find that the room was hotter and had changed from rectangular to circular. I would swear that I was in a different location on a different floor which fed my confusion and although upsetting to me just made my family wonder how much I was in touch with reality. The pillows felt like concrete and were all over the place in the bed. Sometimes I pictured that I was spotlighted like in an operating theater. In my delirium I wasn't sure if I'd had an operation, was having one or was waiting for one.

One thing that had occurred was that my family had confiscated my cell phone to keep me from calling people. They did this to preserve my remaining credibility, because I was just talking nonsense. As my brother put it, I was "way gone". My family was really concerned at this point, since I was not making much sense at all. In addition, one of the consequences of my encephalaphy was the constant shaking of my hands. There would be days where I dropped anything that was handed to me.

So to sum up, I could:

- Carry on conversations with non-existent landscape people. They were all poor poker players. At one point I thought I heard my cell phone ring and not being able to find it carried on a conversation holding the remote control for the television to my ear.
- Drop anything handed to me. Including the remote control or cell phone.
- Fall asleep while people talked to me.
- I could not read (One of my great joys) or concentrate on any subject.
- I could never find the same TV station, even though it seemed to be a simple setup.
- And I could stir the stars, although this was rather fun and magical.

To show me how far I had declined and to test how far I had deteriorated or lost touch, my family would test me by playing cards (Especially cribbage or pinochle) these were games I had played since I was five years old. When I could no longer count cards or move the pegs, they knew I was sinking deeper into my semi-hallucinatory state.

As it was the constant interruptions of sleep patterns began to take its toll on me. With my wife, doctors, and family wanting me to be awake throughout the day and the nursing staff taking vital signs every hour or two, I "began" to get pretty darn surly if someone woke me up. (I'm sure their description of my surliness would include some additional adjectives.) My lack of understanding of my condition also contributed to my anger and confusion. I had hoses, monitors, adhesives, ports and tubes everywhere. I hated them all, and since I didn't really understand their purpose I would remove them when I could.

This usually led to blood all over bedding and the walls. You will be prohibited in most unpleasant ways from removing your tubes. I did learn one secret (save it until you really need it, or they will fix you real good). Since I was hooked into a heart and respiratory monitor, if I thought that I wasn't getting attention by pushing the call button, I would remove these leads. Nothing gets a staffs attention like their monitors flat-lining. Within a very short time of the disconnection I would have staff from everywhere wanting to help. Problem is if you continue to do this, the "little boy who cried wolf" syndrome could cause some serious consequences.

Despite my hallucinatory state, I was still capable of studying the methods and procedures of the hospital. This is a serious topic. I consider myself to be a management professional, who has studied American, European, and Japanese methods for improving service and reducing overall costs. The apparent lack of control between the medical professions and the insurance companies leads to ultimately unhealthy situations. People of the United States have to pay more for much less services. For example I had three doctors all wanting to have blood test performed. Rather than their staff's getting together and getting all of the information from one test, I was poked three different times.   This doesn't seem like much, until you realize that each blood test was costing my insurance company $100 and myself $15. This produced a tripling in costs for no valid reason.

Thus, to sum up, the following areas apply:

- Insurance companies are in business not to pay for services, but to make money.
- Americans rarely take responsibility for their own
- health.
- Doctors and hospitals are deathly afraid of any
- litigation.
- Lawyers (See TV Advertisements) are constantly looking for big bucks or low-hanging fruit to get a quick or extensive payback.

What does all that mean?

- We pay for tests that are completely uncalled for and not necessary.
- We are constantly badgered and awakened to ensure that you won't go 'south". (what do you mean by go south?)
- We pay more for services despite the insurance.
- Doctors rarely treat us as a whole patient.
- Everyone wants us out of the hospital as soon as possible.

A typical situation is the hospital staff inserts an IV, and follows one doctor's orders for drugs and tests, which are then followed up by another doctor wanting similar tests but now the IV is dedicated to the previous doctor's orders. During my first stay in the hospital, I had a total of ten different doctors assigned to me. (These included Infectious disease specialists, liver specialists, and a team of surgeons). They spent more time arguing amongst themselves concerning the correct course of treatment rather than getting me better individual care. I understand that the best medical minds will disagree on causes, drugs and, treatments, but this many rarely led to a consensus. Surprisingly enough I developed amazing relationships with people who did not exist at all, my friends from the paintings. Since these hallucinations "appeared' to be much more concerned whether I lived or died and liked to talk about things other than which needle was going to be poked where, I talked to them long and often. They loved to play poker and many times would give me items that disappeared later, such as magazines, radios, or watches. This was a source of great amusement to me, since no one else could see or hear them. From other points of view, it often appeared I was talking to myself. And, in fact I was.

One day, I was transported with the usual protocol... Can you walk...etc?" They delivered me to a darkened hallway to wait for the previous patient to clear a room where I would be staying. Two extremely efficient nurses installed a "PICC" line that dumped antibiotic and drugs directly into my veins. A "PICC" line is a far more effective way to deliver drugs and antibiotics to a patient. The line is inserted through your upper arm and goes directly to the vena cava. Any compound inserted through the line is rapidly spread throughout your body.

Initial Recovery, Return to work, and Re-infection:

Despite all of this assistance, I began to get better. This was also my first brush with the PT/OT group in the hospital. The Occupational Therapist and Physical Therapist perform valid and essential functions, but they are some of the most arrogant employees in the hospital. They are completely independent of the doctors and nursing staff, make up their own schedules and seem to care less about your personal needs or concerns. I know that they mean well, but it is rare that the best interest of the individual patient enters into their thoughts....I even got pretty sarcastic concerning when to anticipate their appearance. It would always be late in the afternoon, when my energy levels would be at their lowest.

They do perform several fine functions, such as how to use other legs to give you leverage in or out of bed, how to stand up, and how to climb stairs. But during one three day period, they either showed up during a nap or right in the middle of my meal. (The infection specialists had finally won the battle with the surgeons, and I would not have an operation at this time... so I could eat and drink) However, there is nothing like being incredibly hungry, having your food delivered and then having the therapy team show up and have you spend an hour walking. Since there is little to look forward to in the hospital, except for meals, this seemed to be almost a planned torture. They were also not bashful at all about not caring that I had just expended almost all of my energy, they still wanted me to perform like a dancing bear just for them. There was one occasion where I had the nurses, my family and even my doctor tell them that I had just walked down the hallway and ascended a flight of stairs; they refused to believe anyone until I did for them again. I guess it wasn't in my chart or they would have known.

Enough about physical therapists, the occupational therapists want to know:

- How do you plan on returning to work?
- Show me how you put your socks on.
- Do you have an elevated toilet?
- Do you have handles in the shower?
- Do you have a walker?
- Show how you get out of bed.
- What are you going to do to get out of bed, when a trapeze is not available?
- What happens if you fall?
- Show me how you shower.

These are important topics, but not really germane to me at the time. If I were mentally deranged or completely incapacitated, it might be important, but I would be billed $200 per visit for these kinds of questions.

As I mentioned before, I had developed into what the physicians described as "an interesting medical case" (Heaven help me or anyone so designated!) As I mentioned before, the infectious disease doctors eventually won out over all the objections of the surgeons, internists, etc... The infectious disease doctors, were the ones that had wanted the "PICC" line installed. Unfortunately for me, the distance between the exterior entry point and the stanchion for the antibiotics was only about four feet long. This required that I remain for extended periods of time flat on my back and staring at the ceiling with my arm above my head.

Thank god, the antibiotic finally began to attack the septicemia and overcome the infection. Of course the drug of choice by the infectious disease specialists cost $1000 per application. This meant it only cost me $100 per application. But by this time fiscal reasoning was the last thing on my mind. I had reached the point of "Do whatever is necessary to get me out of here!!!!!"

I think that the medical team planned on keeping me for at least another 4-5 days, but a late occurrence finally brought them to my side. The situation caused them to also want me out of there. Late one night, I became very uncomfortable. All of my pillows were on the floor. Luckily or unluckily, I had been placed in isolation. My infection was purported to be dangerous and they did not want it to spread throughout the hospital. Because the hospital was over three hours and a ferry ride from our house, my wife had taken to staying in my room overnight. Many hospitals have an extended windowsill, where people can sit and visit with the patient without bringing in chairs that block nursing access to all of your vital signs. I only had the one bed, so my wife rested and/or slept on the windowsill. She had clothes, a portable DVD player, phone, and some of the comforts of home. Well, she had a few comforts from home.

I was in a bed that was fixed to an bed alarm, so that if I tried to get up, it immediately would sound a beep..beep..beep. Unfortunately, it also would beep if I even adjusted myself in bed. I asked that the alarm be removed, but this was denied. Finally, one of my family members, disconnected the alarm so I could get some sleep. My wife thought that this was a bad idea, and she was eventually proven correct. She was asleep on the windowsill, when I decided to get my pillows which had fallen on the floor. As I slipped down the bed and tried to stand up, she awoke and screamed, "What the hell are you doing?" I immediately tried to back up, but I couldn't maintain my footing what with my weight, weakness and drugged state.

This unbalanced me and since I was unsteady on my feet to begin with, I began to back up precipitously. Each step nearly brought me back to a balanced position, but not quite. Then I hit the laundry bin. (A lightweight structure meant for soiled linens, etc.) Once I hit that, I gave up and I could hear my brain say "You are going down and this is probably going to hurt." I collapsed on the floor, while my wife continued to scream at me. The fall didn't hurt, but I had a plethora of help arrive.

Even the normally sleepy night nurse, could hear the commotion by this time, including the loud thud as I and the laundry bin hit the floor. Now, I mainly had the wind knocked out of me, and will say that I was relatively scared; but I now had to answer the six major questions asked by skilled staff all over the hospital.

What's your name?
Where are you?
Who is the president of the United States?
What is your birthday?
What city are you in....?
What in the hell were you doing?
Who took off the alarm?
At least when the orderly showed up, he added the usual question of "Can you stand up and walk?"

With the assistance of the registered nurse, the licensed practical nurse and two orderlies, I was again plopped back in my bed which I viewed as a prison. But I had the new addition of the stalag 17 guard tower. Any movement on my part brought an immediate and figurative machine gun trained in my direction. Actually it was just an orderly who was stationed in my room for the night.

This did have a surprising effect...It turned the staff into a fully supportive organization geared to getting me out of the hospital as soon as possible. All I needed now was to have the "PICC" line made mobile and get the support of the infectious disease experts for a release from what I had begun to see as a prison. Within one day, I was released, when the infectious disease experts gave a power point to me on how I had responded to treatment. Also, my family decided that I could be coherent long enough to have my conversation with the potential new company (My old company had lost a contract) this company wanted my expertise to help with start up, hiring, and ultimately the running of their maintenance functions.

Within two weeks, I was back to work with two jobs. Although I had always been able to overcome weakness and perform, in retrospect I should have taken more time to heal. I would say that in many cases, most people do not give themselves time to be sick. This is just as true of people with head colds who struggle into work and spread disease to their co-workers. We as a society should be looking into or demanding that sick people get well, before returning to the work environment.

To reiterate the problems with the first hospital:

- The use of shift meetings occur without doctors and do not use the patient charts, but instead use verbal transfer of issues. The use of patient transfer meetings occur without doctors and do not use the patient charts. They instead use verbal transfer of issues. No notes are used and it is common for mistakes previously caught to occur again (Glucose or Acetaminophen in my case).

- The staff had a complete lack of any bedside manner. They did not self-censure their comments about my condition in front of me, nor did they keep me informed of the progress of the disease or treatment.

- The head nurse self prescribed the use of a catheter for an unexplained reason, even after the I questioned whether the doctor had ordered it (Which he had not).

- No one ever thought to explain to the transfer organization (Which is always a separate group of the hospital staff) my condition prior to movement. Nor did the transfer organization ever keep track of existing conditions prior to sending inadequate resources to accomplish their task. In other words a small, often 125 to 140 pound orderly to move a weakened and irritable 300 pound man.

- The OT/PT staff would never provide an advanced schedule, but almost always arrived at the time of the patient's lowest energy level or dinner time to demand performance.

- Since I was awake at night and asleep during the day, no provisions were allowed for my advocates to be in the room when I was awake. We broke several rules by my Wife staying in my room on the windowsill.

- Not only did the TV not work well, no one could explain how the channels could be selected or even changed

Throughout my first stay in the hospital, I was always trying to make contact with my work network for my next work position. Thank God, but my family protected me until I was more coherent by hiding my cell phone. This probably saved many embarrassing incidents, since I could start a conversation with my future employer and then start discussing grape prices in Argentina with my imaginary friends; or even worse talk to the people constantly coming out of the painting. Couple this with playing imaginary poker with people coming out of landscape paintings, and you have a clearer picture.

After six days in the hospital, it was determined that I could walk and was seemingly out of the shadow of death from septicemia. I was sent home with my antibiotics costing $2000 per day, and I was visited by health professionals every other day to take my vital signs. Every morning, my wife would pump my pic line with saline, antibiotics, and heparin. This usually took at least twenty minutes.

As I mentioned before, within the month, I was stupidly back working 50 hours per week and had passed through interviews for selection to the new company. I was to begin working for the new company, while maintaining performance with my old company (Being very careful to avoid any conflict of interest) it was more like me in the old days, where I would work myself into a frazzle. (Stupid.... Duh) I started full time for the new company, and except for antibiotics and pain medications, was performing well. My leg was still dragging, but I could get around with a cane, climb stairs and perform my duties. After two weeks, of working for the new company, my antibiotic prescription was removed. Unfortunately, the source of the infection had not really been identified and handled. Within one week, the infection reasserted itself and I could not walk on the leg again.

1st Operation:

Having been through this once already, I immediately went to see my regular doctor. I was finally listening to my body and I knew that I was sick again. My temperature spiked to above 101 degrees, and my doctor immediately sent me to a new hospital XYZ (closer to home) for admittance. I was admitted Friday and by Monday, my condition had deteriorated enough to require immediate surgery.

A new doctor, the orthopedic surgeon, came in to talk to me and mentioned that it was unusual for any infection to start in the hip and they were looking for the source of the infection. I had had a series of CAT scans and MRI's and the results began to make some sense. The surgeon had noticed that a muscle that ran up next to my colon had a spot on it, so he planned to operate and scrape the hip to remove any infection and check that spot   This spot appeared to be the source of my problem. He had operated to clean out the joint, but also he reached up deep inside my body to check this "hot spot". Nothing like having a doctor find a dark spot inside your belly to wake

Jay E. Morrow

you up to new and potentially disastrous issues. Later that day, during my first operation, he said that when they punctured the spot on the muscle grey, pus had run out.

This was my first introduction to the orthopedic surgeon, although he had once worked on my youngest daughter for a gymnastics accident. He had looked at my daughter and her MRI and clearly stated, "she was too big to be a gymnast". He was just as forthright with me, and of all of the doctors, I learned to trust his opinion implicitly. He was always the kind of guy who gave you the information without adding a lot of sugar coating.

Once again, I had a "PICC" line installed and within a week I was discharged to come home. My wife was given instruction on how to inject the next month. Every morning, my wife or I would inject the antibiotic, and then flush the line with heparin and saline to keep it free flowing and un-clotted. And twice a week; I was visited by a home health nurse that took my vital signs. These visits were interspersed with visits by the physical and occupational therapists. Within three weeks not only was I walking again, but much of my blood work had improved dramatically. My family would visit or call every day to find out how I was feeling and surreptitiously check on my thought processes.

Within the next three weeks, once again, I appeared to be getting better, and my wife had already scheduled to go on a long trip throughout the southwest with her family. So after checking with all of the doctors, she took off for the Grand Canyon and beyond. She made arrangements for friends and family to periodically check on me. I was getting to the point where it was relatively easy for me to get around. I would talk to her almost daily, with reports full of optimism concerning my overall condition. I could almost walk like a normal person with a slight limp. My blood chemistry was improving, with my liver functions returning to low normal range. All my system appeared to have returned to normal. Although I continued to be on a prophylactic series of antibiotics, no infection seemed to be present.

I was still on painkillers and one day I had such a negative reaction that I couldn't move at all without overwhelming pain. This identified to me that painkilling poisoning was both real and present if I overloaded on medication at all. This highlights the dangers of having a confused patient self-medicating themselves.

Septicemia(Again), Osteomylitus & my 2nd Operation:

After weeks of antibiotic therapy, I thought I was heading for a complete recovery. I began to return to my original stress level, but the company for which I was working fired me illegally while I was sick. (They eventually settled out of court). Two weeks later, as I quit the antibiotics, I was beginning to walk normally, when the disease struck again. I remember vaguely several trips to the emergency room, accompanied by my Mother. My wife was in New Mexico.

My Mother is 84 and in better shape than I am, but my 28 year old daughter, my 19 year old daughter and my brother all tried to help. My brother had come up from Eugene, Oregon to give my Mother a rest and attempt to beat me in a few card games like he had when we were kids. I think it was a good time for us to connect on a more meaningful level than we had for a long time. Remember that my wife was in the southwest US and until this time I had been reporting to my wife my overall improvement.

But two days later, I am back in the same medic vehicle, with a whole new set of four strapping youths.

It became more than evident that I continued to have problems. Within a week, I couldn't get up from our chairs and I was again returned to the hospital. My weight had ballooned to the point that we had to have the local medics (four strapping young lads) lift me through our garage and take me to the hospital. Now, keep in mind that I could not walk and I have a history of infection. It is late Friday night, and the hospital administration denies me access to the hospital because my illness is not life threatening. "Excuse me....!!!!" They sent me home. Within a week, I not only couldn't walk, I was close to death again. I entered the hospital on Friday, I found myself scheduled for surgery on Monday.

The orthopedic surgeon found that not only did I now have an infection of the hip joint; I had advance stages of osteoarthritis. During the emergency MRI, the surgeon found a total of three different infection sites. The new operation was designed to scrape the hip and check the source for each of the infections and in a worse place scenario might require the removal of my ball joint.

Now not only could I not walk, but my temperature has risen to 102^0F. After a quick consultation with an infectious disease expert, it was determined that I had VRSA, the worst kind of MRSA (This turned out to be inaccurate). That night my temperature spiked to 106^0 F. The hospital staff put me on a brand new machine that essentially placed an ice cold pad underneath my whole body. Luckily, my temperature reduced to a more manageable 101° F.

My orthopedic surgeon decided on an immediate operation to attempt to clean out the hip joint (They should have installed a zipper, it would have saved everyone a lot of time). He also felt that there was a chance I had osteomylitus (bone infection). Although this possibility was quite low, he needed to warn me (again) that it was possible that I could lose the entire top portion of the femur. Throughout this developing situation, I still managed to keep my sense of humor. One day the head nurse showed up to ask a few questions. She wanted to know what my goals were. I quickly stated "To get the hell out of here." They laughed and wrote it up on my board. Every doctor or nurse saw that on every visit.

Death & Coma:

I went into my second major surgery at a low ebb. I had a major infection, and it might require the potential loss of the use of my leg. Emergency operations are not recommended by anyone, except under the most extreme situations. I remember my temperature spiked to 106^0 and the nursing staff put me on a special emergency equipment that cooled from underneath me. It was bitterly cold, but it did reduce the fever.

I didn't understand completely what happened until months later, but I awakened six days later and discovered that I was in the ICU (Intensive Care Unit) Evidently, I had entered into a hepatic coma while on the table. Tubes had been inserted to help me breathe, feed me, and fill me with antibiotics. A do not remember opening my eyes or any visual information for the next several days. I had strange auditory visions that forced themselves upon me. I was in this coma for six days but I could still hear much of what was going on in my room. This is something to keep in mind when dealing with a comatose patient. I drifted down a long white tunnel, without any guide (Neither Jesus, Buddha, or Mohammed showed up) This phenomena has already been discussed multiple times by other authors, and I would just be treading on old ground. But, along with the white light identified by many dying patients, my first memory after the dreams listed below was my wife and mother reading books to me while I was struggling to return from the coma. But what affected me most were a series of visions. The following still remain as real as ever for me now as when I was comatose.

Vision 1:

I cannot move, but I know that I'm in Alaska, where I was born. It is incredibly dark, and I am in a doughnut shaped space. I am attached by ropes and cannot move more than a few inches. I itch all over, but cannot scratch. I yell but no response is evident for hours. Finally, a servant arrives to tell me to be quiet or they will tightly attach me even more, with ropes that will allow no movement. No one will talk to me, but I am tied down to some structure. (I live in the Northwest, where totem poles are readily evident.) A group of totem spirits is arguing about whether I should live or die. These visionary spirits are representing the side that want me to live and the forces that are trying to kill me. There was a crow, a bear, an eagle, an otter, and an elephant (Some eastern symbols crept in there). I tried to assert myself and weigh in on the side of letting me live. They let it be known that I couldn't tell which side was which, and that I had no role to play at all. Although I did learn to release from the hubris of everyday life and let things happen and change what I valued about myself. As soon as I released from the vision of life as I thought it should be, and relaxed with my predicament. This impacted beyond the Vision and my life has changed considerably since this event. As I returned to another Vision, the last thing I remember was the spirits saying that if I ever returned again, I would die.

Vision 2:

I am sitting at a different floor in the hospital, one floor above my current hospital location. I am included in the survivors from the *HMS Hood*. I wait for hours for other members of the surviving crew to arrive. Even though, I know that only three survivors of the *HMS Hood* survived their meeting with the *Bismarck*. The *HMS Hood* was the pride of the British Navy during the early days of World War II. It had developed an almost mythical quality as the best ship within the British Navy. After the third salvo from the Bismarck, the *HMS Hood* blew up. The dinner plates were all marked with the logo of the English royal family. In my Vision I was alone and could not find any silverware. I called in vain for someone to bring me silverware, but it gradually donned on me that I was alone. In my struggles with this dream I could not get anyone to pay attention to me. In my thrashing I had removed my heart and lung sensors. A surprising amount of attention arrived moments after my sensors flat lined.

Vision 3:

In Shangri-la did Kublai Khan build Xanadu his pleasure palace. To this misquotation of Coleridge, my mind kept returning and ruminating.

I was located in a high tower with a special need for a handkerchief.

This Vision concentrated on the fact that I was in a tower surrounded by light, and it was vitally important that I get someone to help me. This tower was at the end of a tall spire and I was surrounded by spotlights that isolated me from everyone else. This tower was in a hospital, but I was on the very top floor. I was so dry in the throat and mouth that I remember asking for a covering for my mouth. It was so important that I wanted something to hold the handkerchief in place; I couldn't think of anything else other in finding a way to moisten my throat and mouth.

After an extensive search throughout the hospital spire, my wife finally offers a rubber band to hold the cloth in place. I cannot believe that in an entire hospital that more capabilities do not exist for making me comfortable. Once the handkerchief is installed, I thought that my troubles breathing would end and I would finally sleep the night away without struggling to breathe. The installation of the covering had no impact, and my struggles to breathe continued.

Vision 4:

I am in a separate floor of the hospital. I could not get the attention of the night attendants. She and her helpers were studiously ignoring me. I was sure that they were asleep and could not be bothered by me and my petty concerns. I entered into a long discussion with my wife concerning the nature of the family. It was a long discussion concerning sex, duty, and what it means to love. The night nursing staff was studiously ignoring us. Our discussions took all night, which was convenient since neither of us could get the attention of the night nursing staff.

Vision 5:

I am in an empty pool room with wires around my head. I know that I should not touch the wires, but my curiosity gets the better of me. I attempt to remove the most innocuous wires. I hear a voice outside of myself, say don't touch that, but it is too late and they must reinstall the breathing tube. At this point I hear an authoritative voice saying... "Jay, why do you do that?"

You notice that the Visions gradually got more and more real and started to include family and hospital staff. It was like was returning from a deep well and my mind was including more and more actual conditions. Now, why are these dreams important? And this is a point that I cannot stress strongly enough. <u>THE HOSPITAL, THE DOCTORS AND THE STAFF TREAT THE BODY, BUT COMPLETELY IGNORE THE MIND.</u> I want to be very clear on this point. I probably wouldn't have survived without the tremendous efforts expended on my behalf by the team of doctors and nurses dealing with my disease. But, that was not all that I needed at that time. I was dealing with life changing events and they either could not or would not respond in those areas.

As a coma victim, I was aware but unable to communicate. It is critical that you understand that although the hospital staff treats your body, your mind is considered to be the responsibility of your personal advocates. Thus it is vitally important that you have another support staff (friends or family) that understand what is really happening to you. Otherwise, your mind will fill in the gaps with dreams and visions. This is absolutely crucial for any coma patient, where you have absolutely no capacity to obtain information on your own.

My family helped fill in the gaps and assisted me in understanding the processes of renewal that my body was undergoing. My first real and true memory is my Wife reading "Zero Day Threat" and my Mom reading the "Humor of Bennet Cerf" and the "The Life of Charles Lindbergh". By the way, Bennet Cerf has no humor, and my first conscious act was when my Mom asked if she should read more of the <u>Humor of Bennet Cerf</u> (something which from my point of view is non-existent); I indicated to her that I did not want to hear any more of this book. They were the first to let me know that I was in intensive care and that I had been close to death (once again) and was now struggling with pneumonia.

Late one night, a doctor came in and removed the feeding tube. Now keep in mind that this is one of the worst lines to have installed. When they had reinstalled it after my dream of the pool room, it was like the tube went into my brain and I was forced to swallow to get the tube down my throat. To have anything feel like you are swallowing your brain is obviously not a feeling to be sought. Unfortunately, when the LPN came in she noticed that the feeding tube was removed, and the chart had not been annotated. She asked me where I was located and what hospital I was in, both of which I got wrong. I tried to correct my mistakes, but she was Asian American and her English was limited. She was all set to reinstall the line, when I threw a hissy fit and demanded that they call my Mother. I did not know where I was, except that I was restrained with boards attached to my arms. Later I found out that they had tied me to the bed. Luckily, I could remember my Mother's phone number and had them call her. They did not believe me at first, until they checked the phone number and found it to be a real and true. They finally checked with the Doctor and found out that she had indeed removed not only the feeding tube but the breathing tube as well.

Next we have the appearance of a nurse that I called "Captain Crunch". Although at the time I hated her, she had to force me to get better and not just relax into deeper pneumonia. Whenever, I would kind of choke on my own phlegm, she would demand that I cough. I would try my best, but it hurt tremendously to cough in any fashion. For whatever reason, I equated her to a Union Army Captain during the Civil War. In my perspective I thought that she was very mean, but that is what I needed at that time. I did not realize that not only had I had the operation, but that I had stopped breathing on the table. I was placed in the ICU (Intensive Care Unit) under almost continual watch. My wife had returned from her vacation and my family had gathered to support me in any way possible.

By coughing, I would rid myself of the hardened phlegm caused by the operation and its subsequent pneumonia. But at the time, I was sure that I had ghosts of Civil War veterans walking around my room. The visions of the blue army ghosts became ubiquitous for the next few days. Captain Crunch was actually the ICU nurse that was encouraging me in any way possible to cough up the phlegm of the pneumonia and without her, my stay in the ICU could have been disastrous.

Recovery & Rehabilitation:

In addition to the need to breathe, I now had to show that I could swallow and talk, and remain coherent. Until I did so, I was destined to remain in the ICU. I also had to work with physical therapists to show that I had no hand weakness. Time passed with my family in almost constant attention. I thoughtlessly told my wife one day that I did not want to be petted. She had spent almost continual watch and this put her over the edge and led to tears. At the time, I did not know this, and did not learn of it until she felt I was stronger.

My regular doctor had no privileges within the hospital. Because he lacked privileges, a brand new doctor was assigned by the hospital that did not know me nor did I know him. So I was under the care of a new doctor, my infectious disease expert and the orthopedic surgeon. I did experience one additional indignity, when my regular doctors took the day off, and I was placed under the care of a new doctor, who decided that I really needed therapy and testing for a thyroid problem. I had become so frustrated at this point; I chased him from my room saying

"Get the hell out of my room". It does point out that when your one primary doctor finally takes a vacation or a weekend off, leaving you to another doctor who decides that you really are suffering from a thyroid deficiency. It takes major chutzpah from either you or your advocate to say "No". I wish that I could say that this was the end of my story, but it wasn't......

My life changed forever after these events. Whereas before I had always been in control of my emotions, I now would cry over the least provocation, my family and I both think that this was an improvement over the past, but now my emotions lie just below the surface.

I found out later that not only had I quit breathing on the table, the top of my femur, which includes the ball of the joint, had been removed. How I found out was when the MRI staff was taking a picture, they said, "Did you know you have metal in your hip?" Metal in my hip, when did that occur, I wondered? I found out later from the surgeon that he had replaced the joint with a metal free floating bar and the end was a specifically designed cement joint that included impregnated antibiotic. They installed drains that were supposed to drain the operation site of pus. I kept removing the drains at night. They finally sewed the drains into the wound site. I still managed to somehow remove the drains from the site. Needless to say no one ever explained the purpose of those drains, so I can imagine that I just thought them to be an itchy spot.

Back to the course of events, to ensure that they had caught all of the infection, I was scheduled for an MRI, X-ray and ultrasound. Different hospital, but the same flakes worked the MRI equipment. Once again I heard, "Can you stand up and walk?" but now a new topic was added, besides the issue of the metal in the hip, as I lay on the table, they decided that they could not proceed with the imaging until an anesthetist nurse arrived. So I laid spread eagled on the table, waiting for them to locate a nurse. I found that I did not care, since this was the most time I had spent in the hospital without someone coming by to take vital signs.

I fell asleep and awoke to find the MRI staff taking bets on which of my locations were still infected. It ended up being all of them. Only the new operation site was free of infection. The infectious disease doctor made a potential mistake at this point and identified one of the sites as VRSA (the worst form of MRSA-flesh eating bacteria). This required daily reports to the CDC in Atlanta and meant that I had to be isolated. Until I left three months later, the hospital was always gowned and gloved as if I had the "Andromeda Strain". Later on, he admitted that this was probably not the case, but by that time it was too late.

To help control the enormous pain, I had a special unit that allowed me to self-administer painkiller, a type of morphine. What I found was that it turned me into a clock-watcher. I would press the injector and then wait for another 6 minutes to pass and then press it again. I finally asked them to remove this device and to go back to oral painkillers. Although I liked this better, it made me a slave to the nursing staff's schedule. Unfortunately, when they disconnected the painkillers they forgot to reduce the amount of the saline intravenous fluid. I filled up like a balloon to a weight in excess of 300 pounds again. And I could not get any doctor to come see me to reduce the fluid or increase the diuretic. I looked at myself in the mirror one day and could not believe how much weight and volume I had gained. I felt like a water balloon just waiting to burst.

It was at this time that I created Morrow's axioms of the Hospital

Axiom 1: Schedules will be maintained.

Even if they need to wake you up to take vital signs, they will do so, because the Doctor has ordered it to be done. Only one time (a situation I will discuss shortly) was a schedule violated.

Axiom 2: TVs never work.

My first stay in the hospital, I would find a movie that interested me and explore the remaining channels. I could never find the movie again. My second stay in the same hospital was during the Olympics, probably the most covered event ever. I could never find the current Olympic view cast, only the occasional update.

Axiom 3: Attend to Detail

Do not ever try and get a staff's attention during shift changeover, unless you are coughing up a lung. And even then be prepared to wait until they can respond. Now, since I spent over five months of 2008 in the hospital, let's talk about personal comfort. Every bed that I stayed in had something wrong with it. Either the head controls or the foot controls did not work, but even more was the fact that the controls are placed in such a way as to make them almost inaccessible.

Add to this the fact that hospital pillows simply leave more to be desired than normal. They are incredibly flat and foam based. They do not scrunch at all. My neck would begin hurting after only one night. I finally found a way to have the pillows on the bed support each other and still lift my head to a convenient neck angle.

Axiom 4: They will lie to you

After three weeks on a catheter, I finally managed to convince the doctors that it needed to come out. The nursing staff was resistant to this decision. First they tried to convince me that they needed to retrain my bladder, which wasn't true. At last, the agreed and a nurse came in to remove the catheter. I asked if it would hurt, because then I would ask to do it after my dosage of painkillers. The nurse said it might sting a little bit. After she removed it, it was like she tore up my bladder. I said sting was not the right word for it. Her reply was if she told me really how painful it would be, I would be resistant if not impossible to deal with.

I hope that I haven't given you a false impression that everything was perfect in my family. Many times while my wife was traveling, the only people providing support were either my Mother or my youngest daughter. When I would cry about the situation, it was they that held me or talked me through it. It was hardest on my Mother, who watched as her "baby" boy got sicker and sicker. Not only did she help me through it, many times the only relief from the stress for her, was when one of my daughters or my brother took over the care. But to my relief, my wife and I had very many talks to discuss my care and the stresses of which I was subjecting her. These were difficult, but very heartfelt and helped clear the air for a better relationship in the future.

It wasn't until almost a year later when she saw an X-ray of the joint and saw the MRSA special on the Oprah Winfrey show, that she finally understood my inability to recover quickly. In fact, she understood how lucky I was to have received the proper care.

My sense throughout the recovery period was an overwhelming need to be understood. The pain and inability to walk were completely debilitating. The next lesson I learned was that it made no sense not to take the full load of authorized painkillers. If you weren't scheduled to have two at 2:00 AM, it did not help that you only had one at 10:00 PM. You still had to wait until the appropriate time.   The fact that you were in pain meant nothing, except you got an additional question. On a scale of 1-10 please rate your current level of discomfort.

At this time I had been in the hospital from June throughout most of the summer. Luckily, I was introduced to someone who actually provided good information. We called him the biker nurse and he was an LPN. He was the first to advise me that I didn't have to do anything for which I disagreed. This included medications or physical therapy. He also found a small couch for my wife to sleep in so she could stay in the room. Once we had the couch we defended it constantly as staff members would try and remove it.

Each day I would spend in the hospital I would ask what it was going to take to get me out of there. Everyone was concerned that I had not recovered sufficiently to allow me to go home. I had visitors throughout my stay, who I believe were shocked at my appearance. Many times it was difficult to maintain civility and fain interest in events going on outside the hospital. I still could not focus my energies to allow me even the pleasure of reading. This is important for everyone to understand, keep your visits short but come often. Do not overstay your welcome.

I could tell by this time, that my wife was concerned over the cost of my care. It was over $30,000 in personal payments before I was done. This probably meant that my insurance covered somewhere between $400,000 and $500,000.   Insurance companies do not like paying out substantial amounts of cash, so my wife was trying to deal with the insurance issues, while helping prepare my legal case for the illegal termination. I tried my best to assist where I could, but I was driven by the need to get well. I finally asked an old friend, who was a human resource specialist to help my wife understand how insurance companies and their costs worked. Even though we had COBRA, it was not an easy issue to get your arms around. Specially, when hospitals and doctors do not want to hear about your problems, they just want to be paid.

For my entire third stay in the hospital I did not understand what I was still doing in my room. After I was returned from the ICU, I was placed in a regular room. The days seemed to drag on with no end in sight. Later, I learned later that I was still infectious and they were pumping me full of antibiotics and blood to defeat the multiple infection sites. But this also meant that I was not in orthopedics and so did not have a trapeze to assist me in getting out of bed.

I had lost the top of my femur to osteomylitus. As I said before, the surgery to remove the ball joint included an innovative new procedure of putting temporary titanium post with a cement ball impregnated with antibiotics in the hip. After the operation I could not walk or even put my full weight on the joint. I looked for anything to break up my day. Visits from friends, good movies on TV, or even visits from the Doctors were welcome. Usually I did not see my doctors for more than 10 minutes each day. My body was still retaining fluid at an alarming rate, so that my stomach looked like giant sloshing watermelon. I also would have chemicals added to my daily regimen without anyone telling me in advance. So, I would get a new pill and refuse to take it, and the nursing staff would tell me that it had been added by doctor so and so.

Also at this time I was so bored I would look for anything to break up the monotony. The eating of food, watching television, or playing of cards were often the only thing I had to look forward to break this awful situation, I watched videos and did my best to learn how the TV operated. The TV still defeated me, even to the point of trying to find the Olympics.

There is one additional thing that I could not stand; I could not get the doctor's to listen to me. I often would find that drugs had been added to my regimen, without anyone talking to me. For example, I had heparin injected once per day in my stomach. This was my least favorite of several drugs. Invariably, the nurses would check my blood sugar immediately after my meal. This increased my blood sugar and required the nursing staff to inject me with insulin. I desperately wanted to get rid of the retained fluid, but I didn't just want them to give me new drugs without a discussion. This was my first real information concerning how sick I had been and was still probably infected.

Hopefully you have noticed that my tone changed from seeing the humor in most situations, to a much more serious approach to getting out of the hospital. Most of time, hospitals don't have patients stay longer than one week. I was rapidly approaching three months. This meant two things, I was still very sick, but I now had developed a relationship with almost any nurse assigned to my care. I had seen some of them three or four times. Even they began to feel sorry for me, and wanted me to get well as quickly as possible.

At one point, the one doctor that I really trusted (the orthopedic surgeon) stopped by and I made an appointment with him to go completely through my entire chart. He went through my chart and discussed how the infection had progressed and how much hope he placed in the new device he had installed. The cement/antibiotic had been personally prepared for me by the prosthetic company. He felt it was my best chance to eventually be infection free. One thing we did was order a special lift chair that would allow me to easily get to my feet. As usual, the chair arrived about 7 weeks after I had returned home and was relatively useless.

A new entity entered the picture, when a new doctor came on the scene as the Rehabilitation Doctor. Even though I wanted to go home, she had other ideas. The physical therapy staff at the hospital wanted me to stay with them, since I was making great improvements. My wife wanted to make sure that if I fell, I had the means to get back up on my feet. Finally after much deliberation, the Rehab doctor decided I should go to a Rehab facility.

The second hospital:

o The night nurse was not always available, if she was busy with other patients or it was shift change.

o Doctor's care was almost non-existent. Only one time did I spend more than ten minutes per day with a doctor.

o Again, you can forget about getting any sleep. It is vitally important (I Guess) that your vital signs be taken every two hours.

o Hospitals are hot beds of disease and infection, and this is where I received some of my infections. Stay long enough in a hospital and you are almost certain to get a secondary infection.

o Because of the growth of the medical industry, hospitals have expanded in a haphazard fashion that means to get from point A to point B, requires the use of three separate elevators and stops in several hallways to transfer you to the new areas responsibilities.

o If you stay in the hospital for any length of time, your chart will have grown astronomically. Usually this growth is approximately two inches for every week. Although this course of treatment was occasionally consulted by the nursing staff and team of doctors. Most of the time, it is simply used to ensure that you have not the slightest idea of what is in your chart or how that affects your treatment. Unless, you are especially vigilant or aware it is used by all of the nurses to tell you what the doctor ordered, whether he ordered it or not. If I or my advocate didn't catch it, I would receive many different and dangerous prescriptions.

o The bed in this hospital was designed to keep you inside and not allow you to control this aspect of your life.

o TVs never work in the hospital. If they do work it is impossible to figure out the channels.

o The absolute lowest ebb of any patient in the hospital is late at night. This also the time, when services are the least and when your family is not allowed to be around.

o Most of your care in the hospital is provided by a core of dedicated professional nurses. They are mostly well trained and considerate of your feelings. Unfortunately, because of either the hospitals need to reduce expenses or the individual nurse's requirements. This means all of time spent building a rapport with the first team is completely lost and you have to start over again.

Now I met the absolute worst administrator in the hospital, the social worker. She never even attempted to try and understand how my life had changed and my personal desire to get the hell out of the hospital. One of her roles was to help us find a rehabilitation clinic. My insurance company was attempting to find a local site for my usage. Having been designated as a VRSA patient (the worst kind of MRSA) the first locations denied me their facilities. We kept looking further and further afield. The last site was over 2 hours away from my family. At one point they wanted me to move to a clinic on the other side of a body of water requiring us to travel by ferry. This was both costly and was over 2-3 hours away.

The social worker was completely ineffective and could not understand my need to get home (After almost 3 months in a hospital, even Hell sounds better). I had to meet with the social worker, the rehab doctor, the physical therapists and they still could not decide where I should go.

All of the suggested locations were unacceptable to me. My family was helping my mind get through this ordeal. Having them further away made no sense at all to me. We finally found one only ten miles from the house, but the insurance company would not okay its use. Finally I had to supply a check for $5,000 for the facility to take me.

The Rehab Center:

I was taken by wheelchair and van to the new location. Their facility was wonderful, with pleasant rooms that were extra large. They even had a bed available for my wife. The day I moved in, my eldest daughter arrived and soon started to cry. She was in so much pain with an accompanying lack of strength that she could barely move. She said that my disease had brought on an attack of fibromyalgia. She would spend the next four months fighting this disease, before she found a doctor that could help her. (She is currently symptom free)

The food and services here were wonderful. I got to know the entire staff very quickly and to co-opt them to my goals. I did face one final indignity. I was completely filled with fluids with ascites of the stomach, edema of the legs, and most worrisome of all, my testicles grew to enormous size. They were easily 5 to 6 times normal size and began to choke off my capability to urinate. The nursing staff after working on it for over an hour managed to coax my appendage free, and within a few days the testicles returned to almost normal size.

After months of being awakened every other hour, I was trained to rarely ever sleep. The staff got used to me appearing at 5:00 AM in my wheelchair checking things out for the day. After several hours, I would go back to my room where my wife would just be waking up. I will say that the Rehab center was the first and only medical staff that cared about my physical and mental well being. At one point they even allowed me to skip vital signs in the middle of the night to allow me the first good night's rest in three months.

I'd like to say that things went smoothly the rest of the way, but noooo!   My last night in the facility at 1:00AM the trapeze installed on my bed collapsed and landed on my chest. This caused a minor conniption amongst the nursing staff. As they worried that if I had suffered broken ribs, one nurse even said that she didn't think I had any broken ribs. The head nurse said "Only if his luck has changed". They told me they would have a maintenance man look at it in the morning. This is my area of expertise, and I said wrong....You get the maintenance guy in here now on an emergency. He identified that the trapeze had been faultily installed. The nurses sent me to the hospital emergency room. I was examined by an emergency room doctor who called for X-rays and blood tests and a urine analysis. For the life of me I do not understand why a urine analysis was ordered. As the transport guy came up to take me to X-ray, once again the same question arose "Can you walk?

I arrived at X-ray imaging to find a 100 pound nurse who wanted me to hop around and get on the machine. I said I would be happy to if she would find a walker for me. She said, there were no walkers available. By this time, I was beyond being reasonable, since being awakened with a 100 pound piece of equipment on my chest and staying awake over 12 hours. My comments were pithy and to the point. "You mean in this entire hospital there are no walkers?" Ten minutes later she arrived with a brand new walker with the price tag still on it. Of course, the X-rays showed no damage. The final insult was the rehab center tried to bill me for all of the hospital time and tests to show that they were not culpable. (2 months later they accepted the fact that they were at fault, rescinded the bill and covered their costs for the last day)

Seven Months with a Walker:

Now I entered into a long period of waiting while I continued to heal. I could not put my full weight on the post that had been installed, so I used a walker for the next seven months. I also began using both Western and Eastern medicine.

Since I could not put full weight on the post in my hip, I got very good at using a walker. I rarely used a wheelchair, except for at Disneyland where you get immediate benefits (Head of the line privileges). At Disneyland, we went with my oldest daughter and her two twins. And we had a blast. This also highlights an area of great concern to me now, and that is the treatment of handicapped people in many ways. Although they usually give you parking privileges close to the entrance, it is rare to see a bathroom or a restaurant that has put any thought into how to make things easier for you. For example, most chairs, toilets, cars and booths are too low to easily use. Or you find that many businesses are condescending. Grocery stores that are very happy to help you to the parking lot, but fail to keep aisles clear to allow you to shop. Or you find that there is no convenient place to store your walker, but they will hide it for you to avoid affecting other patrons. You may think I am being overly sensitive until you also try and make your way in a world at half speed using artificial supports.

While I was in this recovery phase I took two airplane trips with my wife and family. The first was to Hawaii. As I was passing through security, I noticed that I was being held up. Since it usually took me ten minutes to get my shoes back on this did not greatly distress me, until I saw over 6 TSA security people looking at my bag. Soon they brought in a supervisor, who finally figured out that the object they were examining was a trigger activated tool to pick up items that I had dropped on the floor. The second air trip was to Disneyland. When I checked in, the airline personnel sent me to a holding area to await a wheelchair. The wheelchair never arrived and I missed my flight. The airline was very apologetic, but said it was not their fault since the service was provided by the airport. They put me on the next flight, which now required transferring to another plane in San Francisco, collecting my bags and getting on the final leg home. I arrived after the rest of my family, who were wondering what had happened to me.

At my wife's insistence, I tried an Acupuncture and Wellness clinic that specialized in Chinese medicine. At the time my painkiller load was high; my diabetes was on the edge of control, my legs full of edema, while my stomach continued to have ascites. I met with an expert in Chinese pulse diagnostics. After I told him of the problems I had, he stated that my problem was in the kidneys, but that he could help with all of the above issues. After only three weeks of acupuncture, massage and Chinese herbs, my edema was gone, my ascites was gone, my painkillers had been reduced by half and the diabetes was firmly under control. I had lost over 60 pounds in six weeks. I reached 175 pounds and eventually stabilized at around 185.

I spent the seven months as productively as I could. I had run out of short term disability and began the tedious process of applying for Social Security long term disability. Although I had the full support of my doctor team, they all advised me that the process was difficult and maze-like. I decided to hire Binder and Binder, who was very successful in getting me these long term benefits. Their comments were that if they couldn't get disability for someone, who couldn't walk, had diabetes, cirrhosis of the liver, and anemia, they were in the wrong business.

Eastern Medicine:

One of nice things about Eastern medicine versus Western medicine is eastern medicine concentrates on keeping you well, whereas Western medicine sometimes seems geared to keeping you sick. They also have never made me wait more than five minutes, before I see a professional. The Western doctors seem to never be available. In fact now, you rarely even get to speak with a medical professional, while you leave message after message on the voicemail. This is a new impact in the medical systems. Not only do they not make house calls, they don't even accept a call from you. Their voicemail takes a message and hopefully they get back to you through their medical assistant.

My eastern doctor cured me of many of the issues I had been facing. He and his organization were the first and only group that cared about my physical, mental and EMOTIONAL well being. His analysis of my situation was right on, and his treatments not only made me better, they cured me of many of the issues, such as cirrhosis. I cannot speak more highly of the techniques and staff who helped me finally to be disease free.

I was really looking forward to the installation of a full prosthesis in the hip. Each visit to the orthopedic surgeon, I would push for the operation. Even though I still had concerns based upon dream one, where the totem spirits said if I returned again I might not survive. Finally the surgeon agreed to the operation, I had a series of blood tests, six in the last two weeks prior to the date of the operation. Now, I was scheduled for orientation the week before the operation. I thought that they would show me the rooms, the recovery room, etc. Instead it was devoted entirely to the hospital's need to ensure that we would pay on time. Seemed a little self-serving to call this my orientation.

Next I had gone for nearly seven months with nothing happening, the longest stretch in 2008. I had developed a new doctor relationship with a liver doctor, who felt I was a candidate for a transplant. This did not seem like my best option, since I knew too many people who had this procedure and the drug load is huge and they rarely lasted more than 5 years. I asked the Eastern medicine professional to work on this aspect, and within two months my liver functions had returned to the low normal range. This was the first really good news I had had in a long time. I like the eastern philosophy of treating you before you get sick to preclude the advent of disease. As of this time, two months after the operation, my liver functions are normal, my anemia is gone, my platelet count is up, my diabetes is in control and I feel great. This is all due to the acupuncture, Chinese herbs, and shiatsu massage.

I was contacted by the nursing assistant for the liver doctor, who wanted even more tests. I threw a hissy fit, telling her that I was concentrating on the prosthesis operation and did not want to hear about further blood tests for the liver doctor. Keep in mind that the liver doctor had done nothing except take blood tests and give me hepatitis A and B vaccine. It was the eastern doctor that had concentrated on the improvement of my liver functions.

I finally had had enough and told the nursing assistant that I was not planning on giving another blood sample or even contemplated taking another test one week before the operation. If she needed information she could contact my internist or surgeon for the results of their blood tests. Her comment was "I don't think you understand how hard the doctor is working on making your liver well." This was just too much for me and my comeback was "It is okay to be arrogant but to be arrogant and stupid is not good". At this point she got really huffy and hung up the phone. It illustrates once again the lack of working together to get one blood test that would have all of the required elements for each doctor. Although each blood test was costing me only $15 each, it was an additional $45 I did not want to spend. In addition it was costing my insurance company

$100 time 3 to get the same information they could have got for a third of the price.

Now keep in mind that my emotions were much closer to the surface than in the past.

- o I cried if my wife told me she loved me.
- o I cried when doctors did not see me.
- o I cried at movies like Brian's Song or Cool Runnings.
- o I cried when Barack Obama was elected.

3rd Operation: (Elective)

During my last session with the surgeon prior to the operation, he told me that there was still a 15% chance that the infection was still there and my body had just encapsulated the disease. He saw no evidence of this, but he couldn't discount the possibility. If the infection was still there I would not have a new prosthesis but my existing post would be removed and not replaced. At that point I would be wheelchair bound for the rest of my life. I broke down and cried in my wife's arms. I always knew it was a possibility, but I thought that the percentage would be closer to 5% rather than 15%.

Fortunately, when they entered the hip, they found no infection and eleven months after the ordeal started, I had a brand new titanium, ceramic and HDPE hip. I was on my feet the day of the operation and left the hospital after only a three day stay. My butt looked like a railroad transfer facility with three different major crisscrossing scars. That was okay since usually only my wife would see it. I began the recovery process that week, and was pain free within four weeks. 13 months after the initial incident, I am working on strengthening the muscles in the hip. After all, I had had virtually no exercise for eleven months.

When I first got home, I had several very strange incidents. I would wake up late at night and not know where I was nor even who my wife was. After a week, this disappeared. Five weeks after the operation; I had had no pain, so I quit taking the painkilling drug oxycotin. I would have dreams where I would be on a cruise ship looking for everyone else, but the ship was so large, I got lost over and over again. I decided to eliminate the painkillers from my drug load. Within three days I was in the midst of opiate withdrawal. I hurt everywhere; I had cold sweats, the shakes, everything except the "pink elephants", although I expected them to walk around the corner every minute of this process. Since they might have been the only fun thing about this process, I greatly missed them. It was a good thing I do not keep guns in the house or my head would have been scattered on the bedroom walls. Within two weeks, the worst was over and I could see the good things in life again. I am currently working on the exercise bike 30 minutes each day in addition to walking in the pool ½ mile. I walk in the pool to avoid any development of a neurological limp. I am close to walking without any support, such as a cane.

In May despite many misgivings by my friends and family, I again took a cruise. This time we went to Alaska. I joined the spa, walked a mile in the pool each day and several miles around the ship. For the first time in more than a year:

- o I made love to my wife.
- o Played poker and won a tournament.
- o I went on a cruise again.
- o I ate in fine restaurants.
- o (Surprise) I went on a cruise again

Final Recovery &
What to Expect:

Although I would hope to never go through this experience again, I am glad that I have changed. I hope that the experiences I lived through in this book will help other people go through the process much quicker, with less impact on them and their families. Knowledge is your best weapon. I have boiled down the main points below:

- o Try to get your support group together to discuss coverage. It is important that the load be shared. This reduces the impact to those who love you the best, while ensuring that everyone will see the treatment provided. Many times. my family would not have believed my comments without seeing first-hand the treatment involved.

- o Remove all forms of communication, except through your advocates. This greatly reduces the chances you will say anything inappropriate or to the people coming out of the paintings. Once it clear that you are sane and coherent, your cell phone can be returned to you.

o Despite having good medical insurance, it still cost my family well over $30,000 out of pocket and my insurance paid almost $400,000 in services. I estimate conservatively that $50,000 to $100,000 was unnecessary.

o Keep records from the very beginning. It is incredibly confusing to try and track the payments and bills from the doctors, hospital, anesthesiologists, scanning services, home health, and prescriptions. Tracking every bill and payment is essential to keeping your costs down.

o Don't assume that the bill is final, until you have a chance to talk with the administration. Many times they will reduce your bill after the fact, if the insurance company has paid.

o Have an advocate that can watch out for you when you are not able to do so yourself.

o Understand that hospitals will treat your body, but your mind is not part of their objectives. They will fix your body, but do not consider your mental or emotional state. Ask your family to help out in keeping you stable.

o Watch out for yourself, since no else will. Do not put too much faith in doctors or medical staffs, their goals are different from yours. This can be as simple as demanding to see what they are injecting into you, to asking to see your chart.

o Have your own system of entertainment, this will allow you to ignore the TV. This could be an expensive portable DVD player or CDs borrowed from the local library.

o You will rarely sleep in the hospital, with many long term effects due to the lack of sleep. This ensures that the hospital staff cannot be sued, but is not very comforting after the third time you are awakened during the night. Try to get your doctor to write on your chart to limit the taking of vital signs at night.

o A mixture of eastern and western philosophy appears to offer the best in dealing with both acute and chronic problems. Western doctors are incredibly good at fixing infections or dealing with the removal of acute problems. Eastern doctors are more in tune with keeping you well, after the acute phase is over.

o Eastern philosophy offers the best return on your personal investment. They do not charge for any of their services in the same ball park as western medicine.

o Unnecessary tests not only occur, they almost always happen for no reason other than the doctors wants to completely avoid any chance of being sued. Always ask why.

o Insurance companies did not get rich by paying claims. Concentrate on getting your fair share. Be as abrasive as you wish, they have thick skins.

For readers of this book, I pray that your experience with the hospital is much better than mine. If this book in any way helps you endure the vicissitudes of a major medical situation, please let me know at www.HospitalSurvival Book.com.